DASH DIET COOKBOOK

FOR BEGINNERS

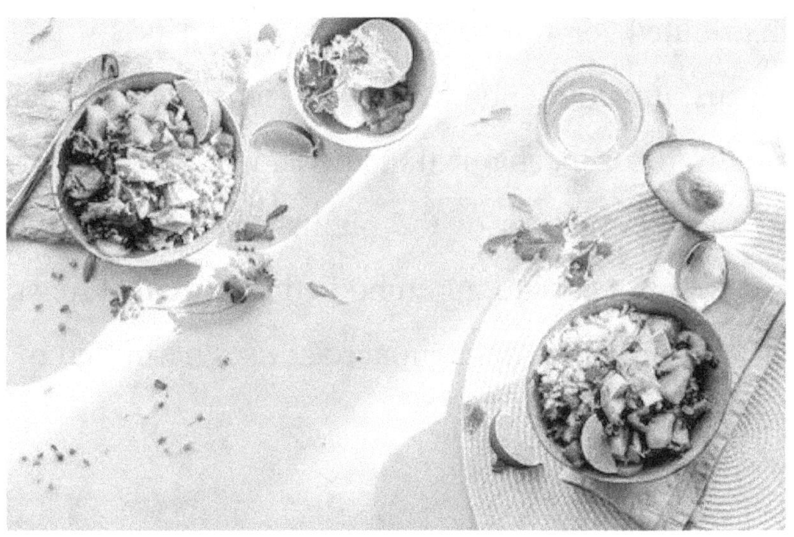

Fast 20 Recipes for Tasty & Nutritious Food,

Treat Yourself to a Healthy Cooking Adventure

Wilbert M. Jensen

OTHER BOOKS BY THE AUTHOR

COOKBOOK FOR COLLEGE GUYS

SMOOTHIES TO LOSE WEIGHT

COOKBOOK FOR DIALYSIS

SMOOTHIES FOR WEIGHT LOSS

DIABETES CAKE RECIPES COOKBOOK

JUICING FOR COLITIS

TABLE OF CONTENT

INTRODUCTION

A middle-aged man who loved big meals, Noah found himself at a loss for what to do after his doctor suggested he change his way of living. Noah was intrigued by the DASH (Dietary Approaches to Stop Hypertension) diet and decided to attempt some cooking using the "DASH Diet Cookbook for Beginners." Flipping through its pages, he saw a world of tasty dishes that would help lower blood pressure and enhance general health.

Noah followed the advice in the cookbook and started eating more nutrient-dense, well-balanced meals instead of his typical high-sodium treats. He played around with colorful salads, lean meats, and inventive vegetable preparations. He used the handbook as a culinary compass, ensuring that he ate mindfully without compromising flavor.

In addition to improving his own health, Noah's dedication to the DASH diet motivated many around him. Noah turned into a live example of the transformational potential of a well-balanced diet as he shared his newly discovered recipes and enthusiasm for healthy living.

DELICIOUS DASH DIET COOKBOOK RECIPES

1. *Grilled Lemon Herb Chicken:*

Chicken breasts

Lemon juice

Olive oil

Garlic powder

Dried oregano

Salt and pepper to taste

Preparation: Marinate chicken in lemon juice, olive oil, garlic powder, oregano, salt, and pepper. Grill until fully cooked.

2. *Quinoa Salad with Chickpeas:*

Quinoa

Chickpeas

Cherry tomatoes

Cucumber

Red onion

Feta cheese

Olive oil

Lemon juice

Preparation: Cook quinoa, mix with chickpeas, tomatoes, cucumber, red onion, and feta. Dress with olive oil and lemon juice.

3. *Salmon and Asparagus Foil Packets*:

Salmon fillets

Asparagus

Lemon slices

Garlic

Dill

Salt and pepper to taste

Preparation: Place salmon on foil, add asparagus, lemon slices, garlic, dill, salt, and pepper. Seal foil and bake until salmon is cooked.

4. *Mango Salsa Chicken:*

Chicken thighs

Mango

Red bell pepper

Red onion

Cilantro

Lime juice

Chili powder

Salt to taste

Preparation: Sear chicken, top with mango salsa (mango, bell pepper, red onion, cilantro, lime juice, chili powder, salt).

5. Vegetable Stir-Fry:

Broccoli

Bell peppers (assorted colors)

Carrots

Snap peas

Tofu

Soy sauce

Ginger

Garlic

Sesame oil

Preparation: Stir-fry veggies, tofu, ginger, and garlic. Add soy sauce and sesame oil for flavor.

6. Greek Salad with Chicken:

Chicken breast

Romaine lettuce

Cherry tomatoes

Cucumber

Red onion

Feta cheese

Kalamata olives

Olive oil

Red wine vinegar

Preparation: Grill chicken, slice, and serve over a bed of lettuce, tomatoes, cucumber, red onion, feta, and olives. Drizzle with olive oil and vinegar.

7. *Black Bean and Vegetable Tacos:*

Black beans

Bell peppers (assorted colors)

Red onion

Avocado

Corn tortillas

Cumin

Paprika

Cilantro

Lime wedges

Preparation: Sauté black beans, peppers, and onion with cumin and paprika. Serve in tortillas, top with avocado, cilantro, and lime.

8. Lemon Garlic Shrimp Skewers:

Shrimp

Lemon zest

Garlic

Olive oil

Paprika

Salt and pepper to taste

Preparation: Marinate shrimp in lemon zest, garlic, olive oil, paprika, salt, and pepper. Skewer and grill until cooked.

9. Sweet Potato and Kale Hash:

Sweet potatoes

Kale

Red onion

Garlic

Olive oil

Paprika

Salt and pepper to taste

Preparation: Sauté sweet potatoes, kale, red onion, and garlic in olive oil. Season with paprika, salt, and pepper.

10. Spinach and Feta Stuffed Chicken Breast:

Chicken breasts

Spinach

Feta cheese

Garlic

Olive oil

Lemon juice

Italian seasoning

Preparation: Butterfly chicken, stuff with a mixture of spinach, feta, garlic, and olive oil. Bake, drizzle with lemon juice and Italian seasoning.

11. Brown Rice and Vegetable Bowl:

Brown rice

Broccoli

Carrots

Edamame

Tofu

Soy sauce

Sesame seeds

Preparation: Cook rice, steam broccoli, carrots, and edamame. Sauté tofu, mix with vegetables, and drizzle with soy sauce. Top with sesame seeds.

12. Turkey and Quinoa Stuffed Peppers:

Bell peppers

Ground turkey

Quinoa

Black beans

Corn

Cumin

Chili powder

Tomato sauce

Preparation: Cook quinoa, brown turkey, mix with quinoa, black beans, corn, cumin, chili powder, and tomato sauce. Stuff peppers and bake.

13. Cauliflower Rice Stir-Fry:

Cauliflower rice

Peas

Carrots

Shrimp

Egg

Soy sauce

Ginger

Garlic

Preparation: Sauté cauliflower rice, peas, carrots, shrimp, egg, ginger, and garlic. Add soy sauce for flavor.

14. Pesto Zucchini Noodles with Cherry Tomatoes:

Zucchini

Cherry tomatoes

Pesto sauce

Parmesan cheese

Preparation: Spiralize zucchini, sauté with cherry tomatoes. Toss with pesto sauce and sprinkle with Parmesan cheese.

15. Mediterranean Lentil Soup:

Lentils

Tomatoes

Carrots

Celery

Onion

Garlic

Vegetable broth

Cumin

Coriander

Lemon juice

Preparation: Sauté onion, garlic, carrots, and celery. Add lentils, tomatoes, vegetable broth, cumin, coriander. Simmer and finish with lemon juice.

16. Cucumber Avocado Salad:

Cucumbers

Avocado

Red onion

Dill

Greek yogurt

Lemon juice

Salt and pepper to taste

Preparation: Dice cucumbers, avocado, and red onion. Mix with dill, Greek yogurt, lemon juice, salt, and pepper.

17. Chicken and Vegetable Kebabs:

Chicken thighs

Bell peppers (assorted colors)

Red onion

Cherry tomatoes

Olive oil

Oregano

Garlic powder

Salt and pepper to taste

Preparation: Marinate chicken in olive oil, oregano, garlic powder, salt, and pepper. Skewer with vegetables and grill.

18. Baked Cod with Lemon and Herbs:

Cod fillets

Lemon slices

Fresh parsley

Olive oil

Garlic

Salt and pepper to taste

Preparation: Place cod on a baking sheet, top with lemon slices, fresh parsley, olive oil, garlic, salt, and pepper. Bake until fish is cooked.

19. Chickpea and Spinach Stew:

Chickpeas

Spinach

Tomatoes

Onion

Garlic

Vegetable broth

Cumin

Paprika

Lemon juice

Preparation: Sauté onion and garlic, add chickpeas, tomatoes, vegetable broth, cumin, paprika. Simmer, then stir in spinach and finish with lemon juice.

20. Blueberry and Almond Smoothie:

Blueberries

Almond milk

Greek yogurt

Almond butter

Honey

Preparation: Blend blueberries, almond milk, Greek yogurt, almond butter, and honey until smooth.

Meal plan

Day 1:

Breakfast: Greek yogurt with berries and a sprinkle of chia seeds.

Lunch: Grilled chicken breast with quinoa and steamed broccoli.

Snack: Carrot sticks with hummus.

Dinner: Baked salmon with a side of brown rice and mixed green salad.

Day 2:

Breakfast: Oatmeal with sliced bananas and a handful of almonds.

Lunch: Turkey and avocado whole-grain wrap with a side of mixed berries.

Snack: Greek yogurt and a small apple.

Dinner: Stir-fried tofu with colorful bell peppers and quinoa.

Day 3:

Breakfast: Whole-grain toast with mashed avocado and poached eggs.

Lunch: Lentil soup with a side of whole-grain crackers and a mixed green salad.

Snack: Cottage cheese with pineapple chunks.

Dinner: Grilled shrimp with brown rice and roasted Brussels sprouts.

Day 4:

Breakfast: Smoothie with spinach, banana, berries, and low-fat milk.

Lunch: Quinoa salad with cherry tomatoes, cucumber, feta cheese, and olive oil dressing.

Snack: Handful of mixed nuts.

Dinner: Baked chicken with sweet potato wedges and steamed asparagus.

Day 5:

Breakfast: Whole-grain pancakes with a topping of mixed berries.

Lunch: Chickpea salad with cherry tomatoes, cucumber, and a light lemon vinaigrette.

Snack: Orange slices with a handful of walnuts.

Dinner: Grilled fish tacos with whole-grain tortillas and coleslaw.

Day 6:

Breakfast: Vegetable omelet with whole-grain toast.

Lunch: Quinoa bowl with black beans, corn, tomatoes, and avocado.

Snack: Celery sticks with peanut butter.

Dinner: Baked cod with quinoa and a side of steamed green beans.

Day 7:

Breakfast: Overnight oats with sliced strawberries and a dollop of Greek yogurt.

Lunch: Turkey and vegetable stir-fry with brown rice.

Snack: Apple slices with a small piece of cheese.

Dinner: Grilled chicken breast with sweet potato mash and sautéed spinach.

CONCLUSION

In the realm of self-care and profound well-being, the DASH Diet Cookbook for Beginners emerges as a beacon of transformative culinary enlightenment. Its pages aren't just a collection of recipes but a testament to the art of nourishing the body and soul. As beginners embark on this gastronomic journey, they uncover a symphony of flavors meticulously composed to not only tantalize taste buds but to heal from within.

Would you like to know about microwave cookbooks? Click here

The cookbook transcends the mundane, introducing a lifestyle that celebrates wholesome choices without compromising on indulgence.

It empowers novices to redefine their relationship with food, showcasing that healthful eating is not a sacrifice but a revelation. With each turn of the page, the cookbook becomes a compass guiding towards a vibrant, energetic, and heart-healthy existence. It's not just about the recipes; it's a narrative of resilience, a manifesto for vitality, and an ode to the profound impact of conscious eating.

The DASH Diet Cookbook for Beginners is more than a guide; it's a profound initiation into a life of wellness and flavor, a journey that transcends the kitchen to sculpt a robust, enduring foundation for a thriving future.

Happy cooking

Contact me here